The 100 Most Powerful Affirmations for Self Esteem

Condition Yourself to Explode With Confidence Whenever Necessary...

Jason Thomas

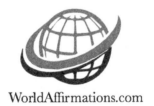

WorldAffirmations.com

You Can Have This Audiobook for FREE!

Just Start Your 30-Day Free Trial with Audible.com.

You Can Cancel Anytime - The Book is Yours to Keep!

Get Your Free Audiobook at Audible.com

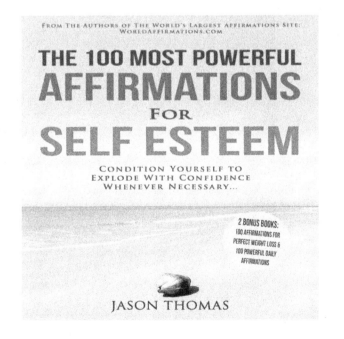

Do You Know **Exactly** How Affirmations Change Lives?

We'd like to give you a **FREE** copy of our book: *Affirmations Will Change Your Life*, available only & exclusively at WorldAffirmations.com.

Affirmations Will Change Your Life gives you step-by-step actions on why you need to use the power of affirmations in your daily life. It's also the precursor to all of WorldAffirmations.com's *Most Powerful Affirmations Series*.

This title is not available on Amazon, iBooks or Nook. It's only available at WorldAffirmations.com.

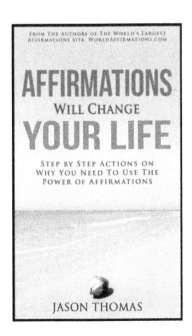

Table of Contents

Introduction

You are now taking the first steps to achieving fulfillment and happiness by becoming the architect of your own reality.

Imagine that with a few moments each day, you could begin the powerful transformation toward complete control of your life simply through affirmations.

You can begin that powerful transformation right now!

You will be able to release all fear and doubt simply because you know that you can. You can utilize this simple, proven technique to regain the lost comforts of joy, love, fulfillment and absolutely any other area of your life you want to improve.

You have the ability to unlock your full inner-potential and achieve your ultimate goals. This is the age-old secret of the financial elite, world-class scholars, and Olympic champions. For example, when you watch the Olympics you'll find one common consistency in all of the champions. Many, if not most, will close their eyes for a moment then clearly visualize & affirm to themselves completing the event flawlessly just before starting. Then they win gold medals, and become champions. These crisp affirmations are used by the most accomplished and fulfilled people in history. That's merely one example of how the real power of affirmation can elevate you above any of life's challenges.

You must believe and repeat affirmations each day, adding a few as you memorize them. If the thoughts and ideas that we affirm are not true in reality, a dynamic tension is created between your perceived reality and your psyche. This presence of dynamic tension causes imbalance between your psyche and perceived reality. Your consciousness will work to get back in tune with the universe to resolve the tension. There are two simple ways to ease this tension. You must work with the universe in order to make your affirmations become true. As you choose to continue affirming, your mind and body will seek to balance this inequality with the universe by transforming your environment to match your declarations of truth. Sooner than later, you will find yourself taking positive and decisive action that you never imagined possible, as your perceptions naturally align with your true reality.

As you begin to attune yourself to the positive energy around you it will become easier and easier to create the world you perceive.

Affirmation isn't intended to make you delude yourself or simply throw a blanket over the negative aspects of your life. The intention is to magnify your focus on the positive reality you desire and the possibility thereof. Affirmation will not force you to get up from your chair and magically start a multi-billion dollar business in a single day. But, affirmation will help you take control of your motivation and release doubt, giving you the power to pave the steps in front of you, as you stride confidently toward your manifesting goals.

You are now striding confidently toward manifesting your goals!

Many affirmations in this book may stick with you or touch you in a special way. Please feel free to take them into your daily life and use them. There is no reason to stick rigidly to the use of any particular set, or to limit your use of them. Find out what works for you. Chances are if it makes you feel positive and empowered, it's working wonders.

These affirmations are for use everywhere. As you begin to use them, you will find yourself remembering certain ones in certain stressful situations. This is your consciousness learning to replace negative patterns with positive affirmation. When you feel this begin to happen, don't worry! The tingling means it's working.

By utilizing these affirmations, you are training your consciousness to work in tandem with the Universe's natural flow of energy. This is how we are naturally designed to function as happy, healthy beings. Unfortunately, the complexity of the world has made it more difficult to find the natural creative harmony we each have inside of us. Negative thinking goes against the larger natural order of the universe, and will unravel along with those who harbor it.

An affirmation is defined as, "A positive, confident, and forceful statement of fact or belief." Anything you think or say is a statement of fact or belief. It's the forceful confidence that gives affirmation its power.

If you want to see positive change now, you'll find the quickest path to fulfillment with affirmation. There is no time to spend on loss, negativity, and defeat when you can be achieving tangible, historically proven results with minimum time and effort invested.

Consider the following your prescription for results.

1.   Review the following list of affirmations in full.

2.   Pick Five to Ten affirmations that powerfully resonate with you.

3.   Repeat several times a day at different intervals. (Minimum Five times a day)

4.   Use anything available to remind you during a busy day: a daily planner, phone alarm, etc.

5.   Do this consistently for Ninety Days.

At the end of these ninety days, you will notice, without doubt, that less and less is happening to you in your life by default. Then you can repeat with the next subject that you wish to make powerful change in your life with.

Enjoy!

The 100 Most Powerful

Affirmations for Self Esteem

I love and accept myself as I am...

I love and respect myself...

I naturally evoke the respect of others...

I let go of any negative images of myself...

I am accepted by others as I am...

I am a unique and wonderful person...

I am a competent and well-rounded person...

I believe in my ability to accomplish my goals...

I am a person who has numerous great qualities...

I can feel how much the people around me love me...

I enjoy spending time with myself...

I am too happy to be alive to wallow in self-pity...

I love and approve of myself...

I will surround myself with people who bring out the best in me...

I make the right choices without hesitation...

I have a great personality...

I trust myself implicitly...

I have as much to offer the world as the next person...

I trust my instincts and intuition to guide my path...

I am always growing and developing into a better person...

I am making wonderful things unfold in my own life...

I am not held back by the mistakes of my past...

I have unlimited ability and potential...

I am proud of my accomplishments and myself...

I am happy to see the person I am becoming...

I am a strong, confident, and attractive person...

I will find hopeful and optimistic approaches to life's obstacles...

I have a deeply rooted respect for myself...

I have valuable thoughts and ideas...

I am fully confident that I can achieve my goals...

I have special talents that only I can offer the world...

I am loved and respected by all of the people in my life...

I am an amazing human being and my life has value...

I am confident and strong...

I am attractive, resourceful, and likable...

I create my reality as I wish it to be...

I am a valuable member of the community...

I love myself unconditionally...

I am flexible and adaptable to change...

I enjoy sharing my success with others...

I work on bettering myself each day with great results...

I radiate friendship and joy to people around me...

I am viewed as a happy and positive person...

I am closer to greater peace and happiness each day...

I have an amazing and fulfilling life...

I have positive expectations of the future...

I will be happy and successful because I deserve it...

I have my own happiness that comes from within...

I have given my life purpose and value...

I am an intelligent and valuable problem solver...

I have an inner strength that others can see radiating...

I have no worries or doubts about my future and myself...

I am able to love others and myself...

I am capable of creating and producing great works...

I will not judge myself for my mistakes...

I am able to choose to live as I wish...

I am receptive to new beliefs and ideas...

I am worthy of receiving love...

I confidently make my own choices in life...

I will be assertive in making my needs known...

I am able to choose happiness regardless of my circumstances...

I am wildly successful in all of my endeavors...

I am a naturally powerful person...

I am flowing with confident positive energy...

I have freed myself from doubt and worry because I am in control...

I am easily liked by everyone I meet...

I approach each new day with a positive sense of adventure...

I have the passion and wisdom to reach any goal I set for myself...

I am confident about all aspects of my personality...

I possess a natural beauty...

I am pleased with the person that I am...

I keep my mind filled with positive thoughts about others and myself...

I naturally attract beauty and positivity in my life...

I am completely comfortable living in my own skin...

I like all the aspects of my body and its appearance...

I see my true inner and outer beauty...

I have an attractive body, mind, and personality...

I naturally feel good about myself...

I have an inner beauty that shines out for others to see...

I will overcome any negative occurrences in my life...

I easily deal with life's challenges gracefully...

I have all the willpower that I need to change my life...

I become more focused on my inner strength each day...

I feel my inner strength grow bigger each day...

I love myself and deserve a good life...

I am naturally strong and enduring...

I respect who I am and others respect me in return...

I am a fun and outgoing person...

I attract people because I am fun to be around...

I am well known for being a fun and likable person...

I am comfortable being myself in the company of others...

I am a good person...

I am worthy of all the happiness I desire to have...

I am naturally confident in my efforts and myself...

I have the power to change myself for the better...

I am able to receive and accept compliments gracefully...

I am too confident to need to prove myself to others...

I am filled with only prosperous and positive thoughts about myself...

I am always proud to have done my best...

I am leading a happy, confident, and fulfilling existence...

The 100 Most Powerful Daily

Affirmations

I am completely fulfilled by who I am...

I will have all the things I need in the right place and time...

I will let the past have no power over what I can accomplish today...

I will remain focused on my goals through hardship...

I believe in the path I have chosen for myself...

I am a good person all the time...

I let go of the habit of criticizing myself...

I am already good enough and I get better each day...

I am happy and comfortable in my own skin...

I have a light that enriches the world around me...

I will unlock the path to success...

I am able to quickly and easily find solutions to my problems...

I have all the intelligence I need to overcome any challenge...

I will bring every situation to the best possible outcome...

I am safe and everything is okay...

I will accept others as they are...

I am loved by my friends and family...

I will follow through to achieving my goals every time...

I trust in my ability to provide for my family and myself...

I am completely in charge of the direction of my future...

I am a magnet for wealth and abundance...

I have a smart and well-arranged plan for my future...

I am able to release worries that drain my positive energy...

I find my work enjoyable and fulfilling...

I attract amazing people into my life...

I am seen as a beautiful and intelligent person...

I am a unique and beautiful member of the world...

I will take time to show people that I care about them...

I will surround myself with people who are good to me...

I am a better person because of the hardships that I overcome...

I have chose to live my life as if it were a gift...

I trust myself to make the best decisions for my own life...

I will find good in even the most difficult situations...

I will replace my anger will love and understanding...

I am able to forgive myself for the past so that I can be a better person today...

I will remain calm and collected in times of great stress...

I make valuable and appreciated contributions to the world around me...

I enjoy the person that I am and the person that I am becoming...

I feel joyful and content right now...

I have fun with everything I do...

I have a great sense of humor...

I rest peacefully and happily when I sleep...

I am successful because I expect to be...

I will learn for all of my mistakes and setbacks...

I will take bold actions in spite of fear...

I am powerful, capable, and confident...

I have the tools to engineer my life as I wish it to be...

I am a beacon of goodness and well-being in the world...

I am in a constant state of massive self-improvement...

I have complete control of my environment...

I will let hardships and obstacles make me a stronger person...

I am not restrained by fear or hesitation...

I exude boldness and confidence...

I am easily able to support and sustain myself...

I adjust to change quickly and easily...

I am confident and secure in the person that I am...

I am achieving all of my dreams and goals...

I quickly become good at things I put any effort into...

I am not limited by preconceptions of my abilities...

I leave no room in my life for worry and fear...

I am loved and appreciated for who I am...

I am a reliable person...

I am at peace with myself as I am...

I will make today a great day...

I have the power over the outcome of every circumstance I enter...

I am reaching all of my goals effortlessly...

I will not be stopped by any obstacles in my path...

I am the one who decides what today will bring me...

I am on a direct path to bigger and better things...

I am naturally attracting power and well-being into my life...

I will make the most of every day...

I will not be swayed by the doubts of others...

I am satisfied with the person see in the mirror...

I am receiving all of the things I need, as I need them...

I give previous mistakes no bearing on future accomplishments...

I will not allow my struggles to distract me from my goals...

I am charting the best possible course for my life...

I am the kind of person who gets things done...

I shine love and light onto all the people I deal with...

I am safe and secure with my life and lifestyle...

I will see each of my endeavors through to successful completion...

I am deeply satisfied by my career...

I am surrounded by people who nurture my well-being...

I am only made even stronger by every struggle I endure...

I am always working toward being a better person than I was yesterday...

I am perceived by others as an intelligent and courageous person...

I have set a clear path to achieving my goals...

I will maintain my already set path to success...

I am not afraid to welcome challenges...

I make the right decisions for my life consistently...

I am going out into the world to have an amazing day...

I will reach the days end much closer to my goals...

I will realize my vision of what today will bring me...

I am radiating positive energy into my day...

I will not take no for an answer today...

I am as smart and capable as anyone I know...

I can envision my goals being accomplished and fulfill that vision...

I am the reason that other people will have a good day today...

I am easily able to communicate with any person I meet...

I am in charge of what happens today...

The 100 Most Powerful

Affirmations for Perfect & Healthy

Weight Loss

I weigh exactly what I choose to weigh...

I am at a healthy weight...

I feel extremely healthy and vibrant...

I only eat food for vitality...

I only eat food for longevity...

I only eat food for maximum energy...

I exercise for stamina and to maintain a healthy weight...

I love to exercise and eat healthy food...

I am most disciplined when it comes to portion control...

I believe in myself and have full control over my choices...

I choose to feel good about my body...

I choose everyday to eat green vegetables...

I perform an exercise program that truly challenges me...

I love eating healthy food...

I love being fit and healthy...

I love how I feel at such a healthy weight...

I write down my health goals to be reviewed every day...

I take massive action on my health goals...

I decrease my intake of toxic foods every single day...

I am what I put in my body, therefore I choose healthy food...

I am so grateful for my healthy weight & newfound energy...

I step on the scale and see the weight I desire...

I choose to feel good and make healthy lifestyle choices...

I let nobody take responsibility for my life but me...

I understand how to lose weight, & I must take action now...

I will weigh what I desire, but I need to get started now...

I eat what I choose, not what others influence me too...

I am proud of who I am...

I feel like a million bucks...

I am exercising every single day...

I feel that exercise is fun, and I feel amazing...

I believe in myself when I set a goal...

I find Fat loss becomes easier and easier...

I feel incredibly strong after I exercise...

I choose to feel strong and energetic...

I have no problem attaining my ideal weight...

I find losing weight is easy for me...

I exercise discipline when it comes to my health...

I am my perfect weight...

I have intense focus on manifesting the goals I set...

I have laser focus on my health, & I take action...

I take full responsibility for my choices and results...

I feel sexy...

I love my body and take excellent care of it...

I love feeling strong & that nothing will stop me...

I love the way I feel, and my body is in balance...

I will only eat foods that will make me feel energetic...

I stay far away from sugar, alcohol and other toxins...

I drink a full cup of water before every meal...

I stay hydrated throughout everyday...

I am fully aware how the foods I eat affect my physique...

I am an incredibly strong individual...

I feel incredibly attractive & love myself...

I have a stomach that is flat and healthy looking...

I have no guilt about my body and food...

I love eating healthy foods...

I hate having to eat sugar and fatty foods...

I have a metabolism that works to keep me healthy...

I will provide my body the fuel it needs to be healthy...

I am incredibly grateful for the body I have...

I am so happy right now, that I can't help but smile...

I love helping my body heal and feel amazing...

I control my thoughts, and I control my weight...

I control my thoughts, and I control the food I eat...

I control my thoughts, and I control the exercise I perform...

I control my thoughts, and I control how I feel...

I am confident with my body...

I am full of confidence...

I have zero doubt in myself...

I spend 15 minutes planning my day to include exercise...

I take small steps that lead to massive change...

I must to move more to lose weight...

I must eat healthier to feel great...

I focus on feeling good about myself...

I focus on the weight that I will feel great at...

I am committed to maintaining a healthy lifestyle...

I love feeling incredibly strong...

I know that no one will do this for me...

I am incredibly clear about what I want...

I am passionate about feeling healthy...

I can and will stick to my exercise regime...

I love providing healthy nutrients to my body...

I love providing healthy nutrients to the organs in my body...

I love providing healthy nutrients to the cells in my body...

I only eat food that will make me look amazing...

I resist temptations of food that destructs my body...

I maintain a healthy lifestyle ongoing...

I feel good when I exercise...

I give thanks everyday for my health...

I help my body become the vision that I desire...

I give thanks for a healthy heart, brain & all vital organs...

I challenge myself every single day...

I love getting out of my comfort zone...

I only eat foods today that will maintain my desired weight...

I have a perfectly conditioned body and mind...

I am a beautiful and fit human being...

I see the person I desire to be in the mirror everyday...

I know losing weight is easier than gaining weight...

I am so thankful for every part of me...

I know that only applied knowledge has value...

Thank You!

I want to sincerely thank you for reading this book!

Let me finish though by saying the work isn't done here. These must be put to use repetitively, and on a daily basis to see changes in your life.

Remember to follow the ninety-day plan outlined in the introduction to maximize your results.

Can I ask you for a very quick favor? Can you leave a review on our Amazon.com detail page to tell us about your progress and how you enjoyed the book?

We take the time to go over each review personally, and your feedback in invaluable to us as writers, and others that wish to see the same change in their lives as you:)

Thank You!

You Can Have This Audiobook for FREE!

Just Start Your 30-Day Free Trial with Audible.com.

You Can Cancel Anytime - The Book is Yours to Keep!

Get Your Free Audiobook at Audible.com

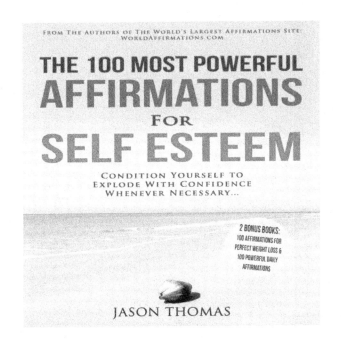